Aromatherapy

The Science of Healing and Relaxation

I0419742

RON KNESS

Table of Contents

How Stress and Anxiety Affect the Body

Stress and anxiety reflect the reaction of the body and the mind when over stimulated. Stress tends to reflect the physical responses of the body when coping with daily pressures, physical labor, a high-paced work environment, toxic relationships, and financial and emotional responsibilities, which exceed a person's ability to cope or manage.

Anxiety emerges as a mental and emotional response to the same types of pressure. This is not to say anxiety does not cause physical responses as well. The mind and the body share a causal and reciprocal connection.

The results of The American Psychological Association's 2010 Stress in America survey showed that nearly 75% of Americans who responded to the survey believe their stress levels to be so high that they feel unhealthy.

Stress and anxiety exist on a spectrum of intensity and expression. Some people experience physical symptoms without the accompanying anxiety. Other individuals experience high levels of anxiety while exhibiting mild or no physical symptoms. In some cases, an individual experiences a mixture of stress and anxiety symptoms of varying intensity.

Stress symptoms include:

- Accelerated Heartbeat
- Headaches

- Perspiration Especially On The Palms

- Dry Mouth

- Upset Stomach

- Stomach Ache

- Tense Muscles Which May Ache Or Tremble

- Breathing Difficulties

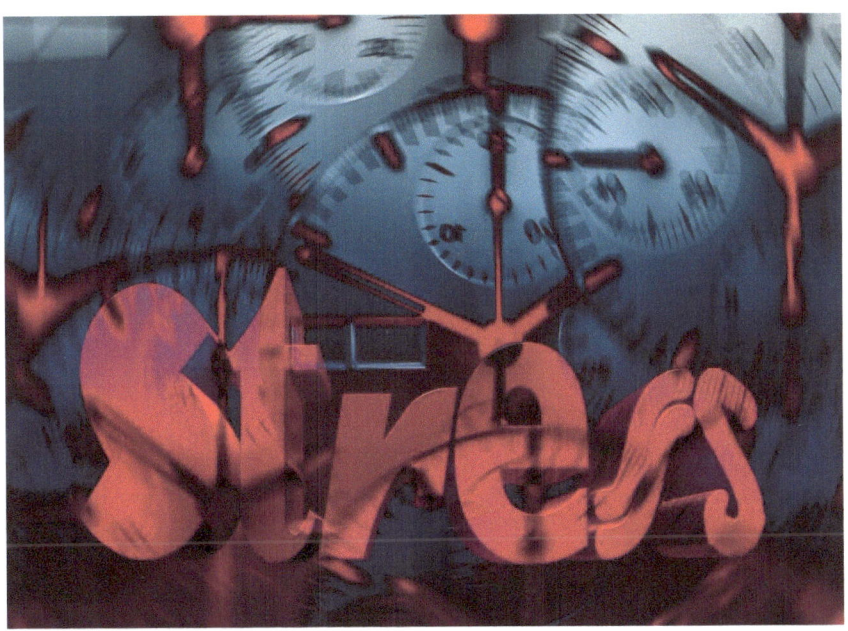

Mental and emotional symptoms accompany stress as well:

- Fatigue

- Insomnia

- Irritability

- Lack of Concentration

- Mental And Emotional Strain

The term anxiety covers a group of mental illnesses referred to as anxiety disorders. Web MD defines four types of anxiety disorders: panic disorder, social anxiety disorder, phobias, and generalized anxiety disorders.

- **Panic disorder:** A person experiences feelings of fear and terror without warning and without apparent cause with unpredictable frequency.

- **Social anxiety disorder:** A person experiences debilitating levels of worry in daily social interactions. They typically fear judgment or failure to meet expectations in these situations.

- **Phobias:** Phobias are specific fears of things, places, or situations, which exceed the level of simple nervousness. Common phobias include the fear of heights, spiders or other insects and flying.

- **Generalized anxiety disorder:** This type of anxiety is characterized by ongoing levels of tension or fear with no specific focus. The level of fear and tension far exceeds the person's circumstances or what would be considered reasonable. In addition, there may be no apparent cause for the fear.

The physical symptoms, which accompany anxiety, share similarities with those associated with stress and include:

- Dry Mouth

- Accelerated and/or Erratic Heart Rate

- Heavy Perspiration Localized To Hands And Feet

- Nausea

- Loss Of Balance And Equilibrium

- Cold Hands and/or Feet

- Fidgeting Or Other Restless Movements

- Tense Muscles

- Difficulty Breathing

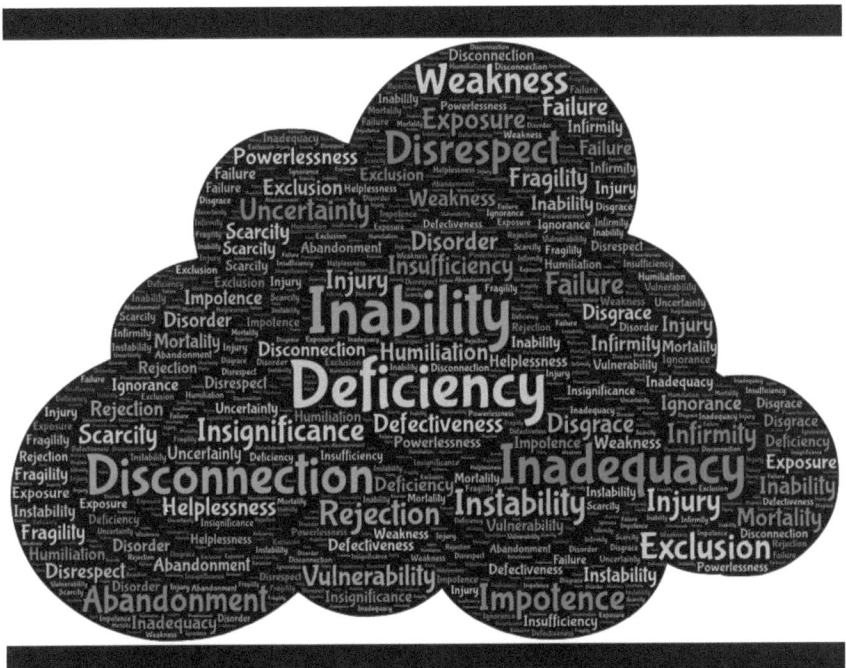

While a person may develop a stress related anxiety disorder, other causes trigger the condition as well. The brain may not regulate the areas controlling fear and emotion appropriately. Certain anxiety orders reflect a problem with links between memories associated with strong emotions.

Anxiety disorders also develop in people with a genetic predisposition for them; some disorders run in families. People with no family history of anxiety disorder sometimes develop it as a result of brain structure changes caused by prolonged stress, traumatic or other significant events.

Anxiety's mental symptoms include:

- Insomnia

- Uneasiness, Fear And Panic

- Inability To Be Calm (High-Strung)

- Tingling Or Numbness In The Hands and/or Feet

Stress and anxiety can become debilitating if left unmanaged. If a person experiences one or more of the symptoms associated with stress and anxiety on a regular basis, it becomes advisable to seek the counsel of a qualified medical professional. A qualified doctor can recommend appropriate clinical treatments and alternative therapies as necessary.

Counter Stress with a Relaxation Technique

When humans encounter a life-threatening situation, a surge of stress hormones prepares us to fight or to flee, an automatic fight-or-flight response of the sympathetic nervous system. This response results in a pounding heartbeat, tensing muscles and a state of high alert.

Unfortunately, people activate this fight-or-flight response every day and several times per day because of non-life threating situations, but simply because of everyday stressors.

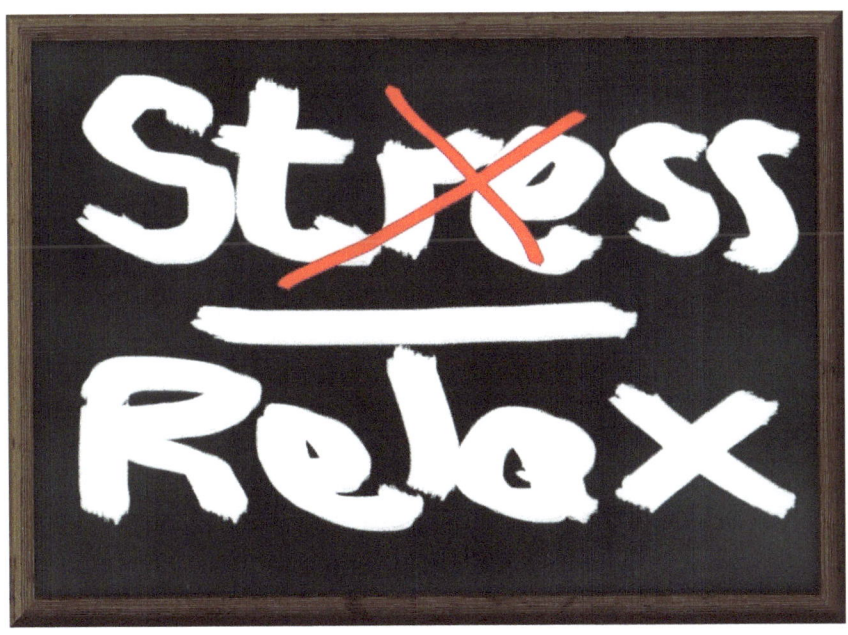

Traffic, being too busy, long lines at the store, bad customer service, take your pick, as all of these stressors flood our body with stress hormones and take their toll. Over the long run, chronic stress leads to high blood pressure, an increase in belly fat, increased heart rate, muscle tension, headaches, insomnia, and other serious health conditions.

The body has an opposite response system called the relaxation response. It occurs when the parasympathetic nervous system is activated.

The physiological effects are almost the complete opposite of those associated with the fight or flight response and true relaxation occurs when the body attains a state of mental and physical equilibrium.

A person experiencing the relaxation response presents:

- An even breathing pattern and heartbeat and blood pressure drops as circulation returns to normal sending blood throughout the extremities and into the digestive system which receives less blood supply during fight or flight situations.
- The mind is calm and the ability to concentrate increases exponentially.
- In physical terms, a relaxed state is characterized by a steady, even breathing pattern, a steady heartbeat, and the absence of muscle tension.
- The emotions are stable, peaceful, and unconflicted.

True relaxation allows the body and mind to shed the effects of the fight or flight response and triggers the relaxation response.

Activities For Relaxation

Yoga, massage, tai chi, progressive relaxation, deep breathing, meditation, and aromatherapy are some of the best alternative activities available to elicit the relaxation response. Each of these activities calms the body and allows the mind to become quiet if not completely still.

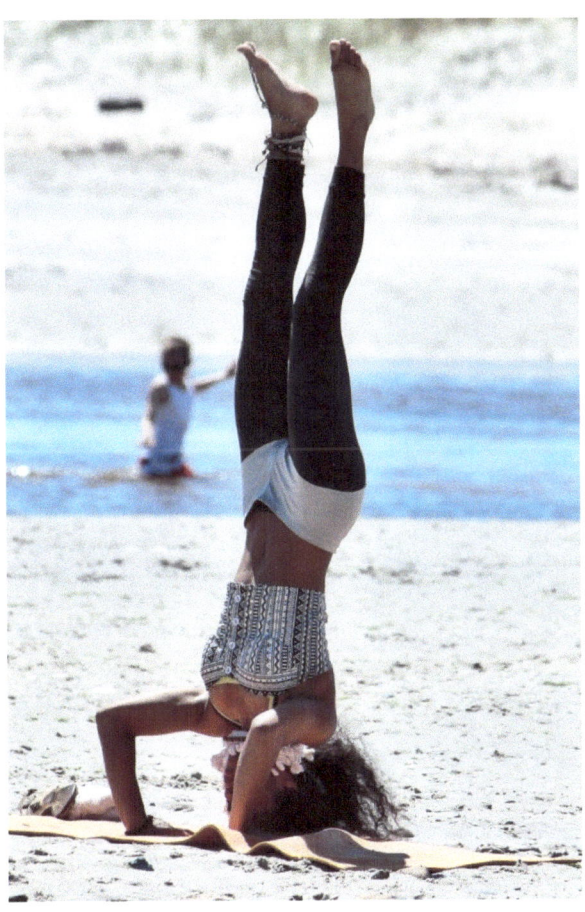

It is vital for everyone to participate in relaxation inducing activities on a regular basis to counteract everyday stress. However, it is even more important for those who suffer from chronic stress to avoid the serious health consequences that can result from unchecked long-term stress.

Stress and Its Physical Effects

The long-term effects of stress and anxiety on the body are detrimental and cumulative. The disease, mental and emotional issues associated with stress and anxiety manifest following prolonged states of chronic stress and the inability to access a relaxed state regularly. Here a distinction must be made between taking a break and genuine relaxation.

When one takes a break, they may fill it with other activities, which bring their own forms of stress. For example, many people express the sentiment of being more tired after a vacation than before they left. This reflects the fact that many vacations are full of activities--not to mention the stressful effects of travel. Therefore, a person trades one set of stressors for a new set of "fun" stressors.

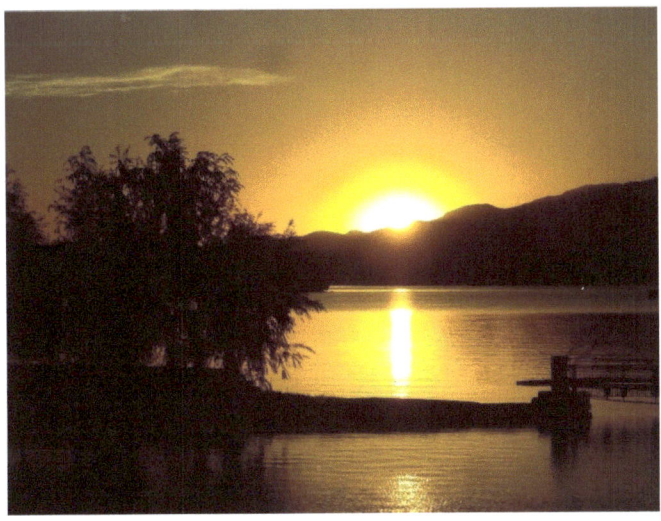

Over stimulation triggers the bodies fight or flight response in the sympathetic nervous system. Fight or flight causes the body to prepare to take action to protect itself by defending or fleeing. The fight or flight response creates a domino effect of physiological and mental responses.

The body prepares to ward off and attack or run quickly by increasing the heart rate and blood pressure, tensing the muscles in preparation for use and sending adrenaline throughout the system. Adrenal hormones released during the response boost strength and speed for short periods of time. The breath quickens and the mind is agitated and difficult to focus on anything other than evading the perceived threat.

Remaining in a chronic state of stress related arousal:

- Wears Down The Immune System
- Causes High Blood Pressure
- Increases Insulin Resistance
- Negatively Impacts Digestion And Assimilation
- Leads To Chronic Fatigue
- Contributes To Poor Decision Making And Indecisiveness
- Prohibits Mental Clarity And Emotional Stability

Americans spend a great deal of time and money treating their inability to relax. According to the Anxiety and Depression Association America (ADAA), 40 million people in the US alone are affected by some type of anxiety disorder. Of the 18% of the population affected by anxiety disorders, only one-third access treatment.

The medical cost of treating anxiety disorders nationally is approximately $42 billion a year. Over half of those costs derive from people seeking medical attention repeatedly for physical symptoms associated with undiagnosed anxiety.

According to a recent paper by economists Dan Hamermesh and Elena Stancanelli, Americans work longer hours, later into the night and more on weekends than their peers in other industrialized nations.

A U.S. worker averages 47 hours of job related activity per week. This level of work has reached the point of diminishing returns according to Hamermesh. People work more at the cost of their social life and their health.

Stress and Its Mental Effects

A person's mood is comprised of the overall tenor of their mental and emotional state. It signifies the way a person feels at a given point in time, happy, sad, content, angry, and calm, upset, or agitated and so forth. Since moods are subjective, people tend to exhibit natural affinities for positive or negative mental and emotional states. Some people exhibit more positive responses, like optimism and contentment, even when in negative circumstances.

Others exhibit more negative responses, like pessimism and worry, no matter how positive their situation. The subjectivity of moods presents a silver lining for people who suffer from stress and anxiety; they can be taught how to moderate their moods to be more positive.

Stress and Mood

A stressed person more often than not exhibits signs of mental distress. They may be irritable and short with people, coworkers, friends, and loved ones.

Depression is closely linked to stress and anxiety, so depression, and a lack of motivation may eventually emerge during states of prolonged stress. Their ability to focus on tasks, plan for the day and the future as well as general decision-making abilities may begin to erode because of prolonged stress. A stressed person appears to vacillate between anger, fear, worry, and general agitation.

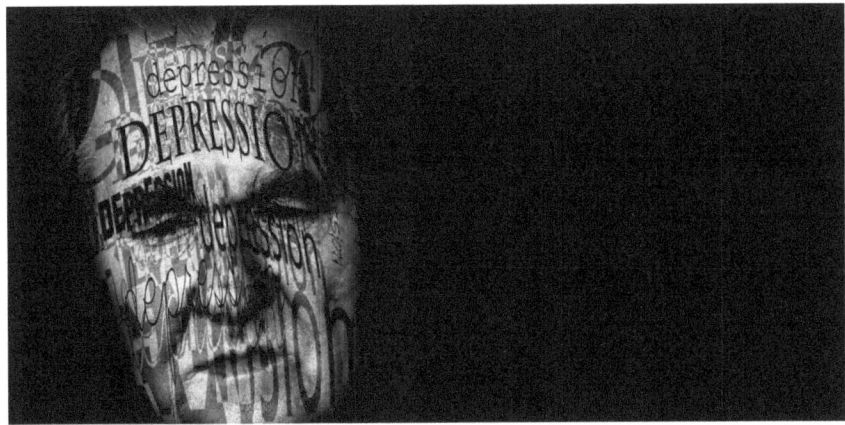

Science is beginning to understand what happens to the brain during stress and depression, which generally follows after prolonged exposure. Depression causes neurogenesis, the generation of new brain cells to slow. It also contributes to a decrease in brain volume called brain atrophy; the rate at which new brain cells generate fails to keep pace with the loss of cells and the cellular shrinkage taking place.

The areas most affected are those related to the emotions, memory and learning. The cells of the brain in these areas appear to shrink rather than die off outright. These results indicate a potential for cellular recovery, a reversal of the condition.

When a person relaxes, their mind calms and their emotions stabilize. They are able to think through situations and modulate their emotional responses. Content is the best description for the mood of a person experiencing a calm mind.

As with stress, the brain exhibits certain responses when calm. These responses or signals, which activate the relaxation response, are tied to the vagus nerve.

The vagus nerve connects the brain to most of the body's major organs. It tells the brain how the body is doing.

Meditation, mindfulness practices, and deep breathing are simple methods to activate the vagus nerve and its calming effects. These practices teach the body what to do to induce a relaxed state.

As the body relaxes, the vagus nerve ferries this information to the brain, which induces a feeling of calm and well-being. A positive mind-body loop is created calming the body and the mind and activating the associated positive physiological effects, lower blood pressure, improved circulation, increased energy, and improved mental focus.

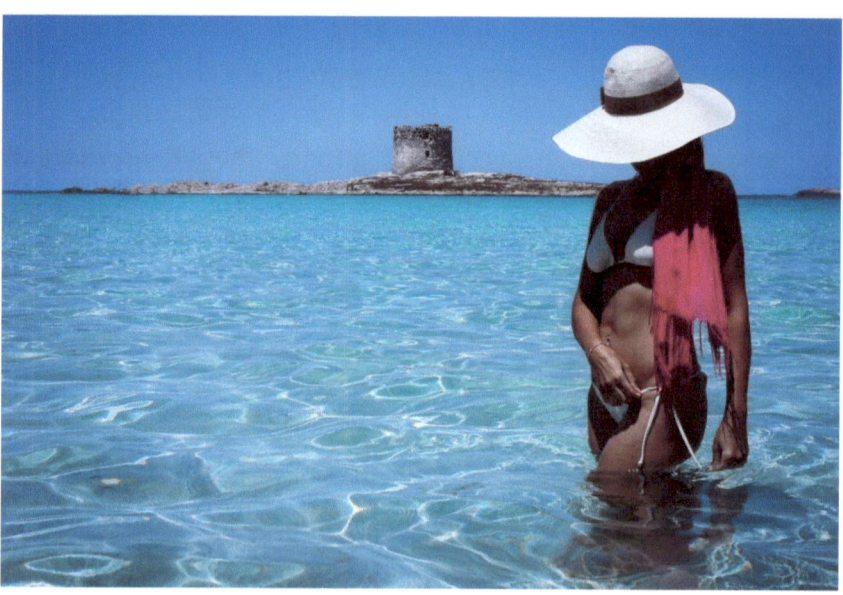

Aromatherapy to the Rescue!

Aromatherapy is an ancient practice, which uses distilled and concentrated plant oils, essential oils, to treat physical and mental ailments. The practice works so well because it taps into the olfactory system, the group of organs and tissues associated with the sense of smell. The structure of the system, the nose, nasal passages and olfactory mucosa lining them, sit in close proximity to the brain.

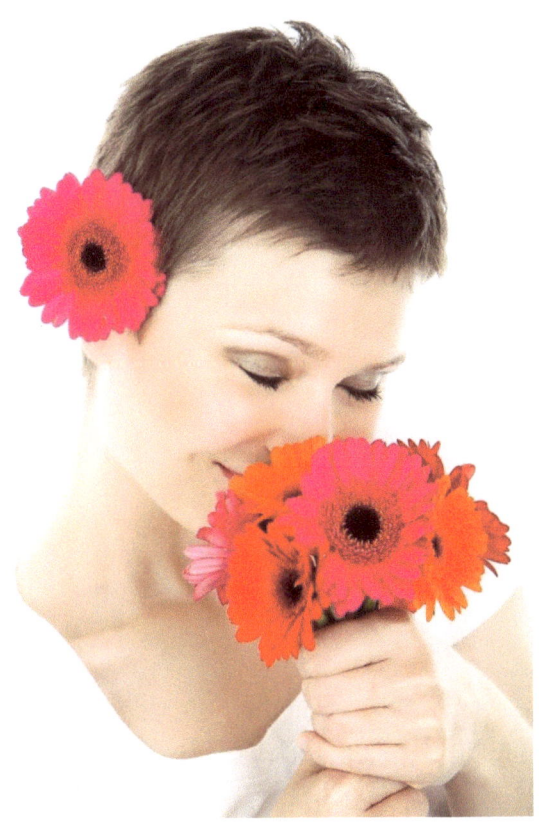

The olfactory system also shares an almost immediate connection with the limbic system. The limbic system controls the parts of the brain related to memory, emotions, breathing, heart rate, and digestion.

Aromatherapy uses essential oils that have the ability to almost immediately access the major systems of the body. The strong connection between the sense of smell, the brain, and specifically the limbic system make this possible. When the vaporized molecules of an essential oil enter the nasal passages, they prompt the brain to send certain signals to the body, which have a healing effect.

How Essential Oils Work

Essential oils are natural oils obtained through the process of distillation and having the characteristic fragrance of the plant or other source from which it is extracted.

Essential oils may be used as inhalants, not the oil itself only the scent, or applied to the body diluted in a carrier oil, lotion, cream or gel. Oils can be selected and used individually or as part of synergistic blends.

Each essential oil possesses characteristics, which make it most effective for treating certain physical conditions and emotional states. A blend of oils imparts a blend of therapeutic results. The results depend on the types of oils used and their concentration in the blend.

Oils should be selected based on their therapeutic properties and if blended combining complementary scents, for example:

- Lavender promotes calm and relieves muscle aches.

- Citrus oils, orange, lemon and grapefruit, offer bright energizing and uplifting scents, which counteract depression.

- Fennel, clove, and thyme oil combat inflammation.

- If a person suffers from arthritis, a blend of lavender and fennel oils might be appropriate.

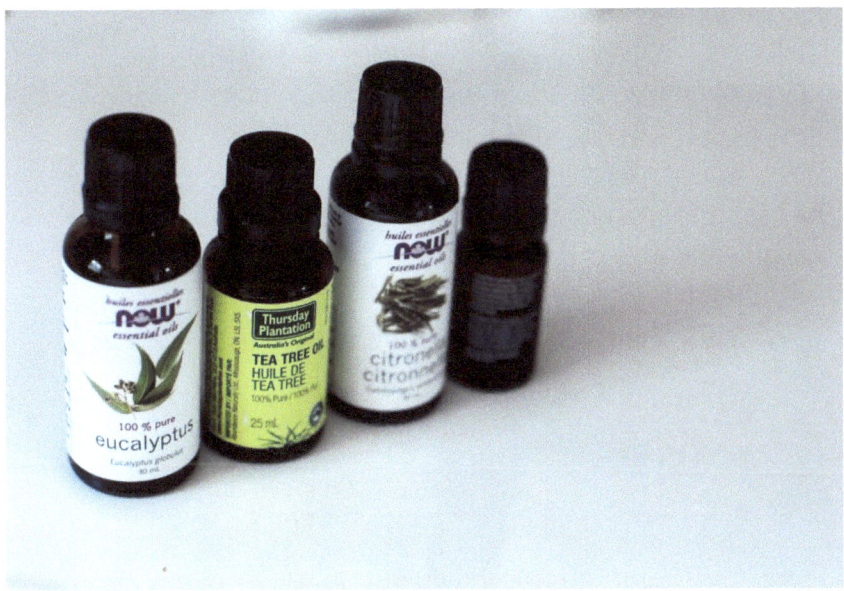

As with all remedies, contraindications and allergies must be considered before making a final selection.

To Relax Use Aromatherapy

When selecting essential oils to use for relaxation and mood adjustment, it helps to understand the desired change in mood. If a person is tired, the desired outcome is to energize their body while calming the mind. If a person suffers from irritability, the desired outcome is to calm them and induce a sense of well-being. The appropriate selection of oils helps these changes to occur.

The following oils may be used alone or in combination with the other oils listed as well as some, which are not part of this list. Keep in mind blends should contain a complementary mix of oils both in scent and treatment characteristics.

The essential oils recommended for relaxation and mood adjustment are:

- Basil: improves mental focus and relieves physical aches
- Citrus oils: (orange, lemon or grapefruit)--uplifting and energizing
- Frankincense: improves concentration and mental clarity
- Geranium: calming and uplifting
- Jasmine: uplifting
- Lavender: balancing, calming and may help relieve insomnia
- Peppermint: mental clarity
- Petitgrain: energizing and uplifting

- Vetiver: has a grounding, calming and stabilizing effect on the psyche

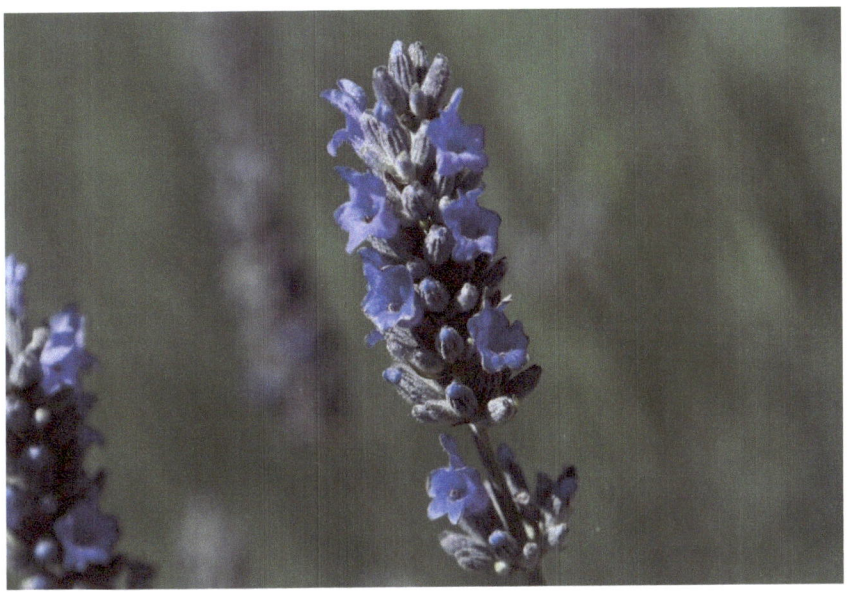

This list is by no means exhaustive, especially when you consider the endless blend possibilities.

Essential Oils – The Science Behind Aromatherapy

When selecting oils to combat anxiety and stress, choose oils with relaxing, calming, and uplifting properties. The oils should soothe while shifting the awareness in a way that grounds and replenishes the constitution of the person being treated. The scents that work best for anxiety and stress relief tend to have light and bright floral, citrus, or woodsy scents.

The following oils may be used alone or in combination with the other oils listed as well as others that are not part of this list. Keep in mind blends should contain a complementary mix of oils in both scent and therapeutic characteristics.

The essential oils recommended for relaxation and mood adjustment may be blended with those recommended for managing stress and anxiety. Many of them are complementary scents with complementary therapeutic qualities.

15 Essential Oils For Relaxation

- **Bergamot**: calming, alleviates depression, anxiety and stress. **Blends with:** jasmine, juniper, chamomile, cypress, ylang ylang, eucalyptus, geranium, lavender, lemon, palmarosa, and patchouli.
- **Lavender**: alleviates stress, anxiety, promotes relaxation and calm. **Blends With:** most oils, especially good with citrus oils, chamomile, and clary sage.

- **Roman Chamomile:** relaxing and rebuilding. **Blends with:** Rose, lavender, rose, clary sage, and geranium.
- **Clary Sage:** relieves fatigue and stress. **Blends with:** bay, geranium, grapefruit, jasmine, juniper, bergamot, black pepper, cardamom, mandarin, patchouli, petitgrain, pine, rose, cedarwood, chamomile, coriander, cypress, frankincense, lavender, lemon balm, lime, sandalwood and tea tree.
- **Mandarin:** lowers blood pressure. **Blends with:** clary sage, vetiver, sandalwood, rose, jasmine, lavender, ylang ylang, and citrus oils.
- **Neroli:** improves mood; alleviates insomnia and stress. **Blends with:** clary sage, coriander, lemon, mandarin, myrrh, orange, frankincense, geranium, ginger, chamomile, grapefruit, jasmine, juniper, lavender, palmarosa, petitgrain, rose, sandalwood, and ylang ylang.
- **Rose:** alleviates depression and stress. **Blends with:** cypress, frankincense, juniper, citrus oils, cedarwood, clary sage, patchouli, pine, rosewood, and sandalwood
- **Sandalwood:** calming and relieves stress and depression. **Blends with:** mandarin, myrrh, patchouli, cypress, frankincense, lemon, spruce, and ylang ylang.

- **Ylang-ylang:** relieves anxiety, depression, and stress. **Blends with:** sandalwood, anise, chamomile, cumin, bergamot, geranium, grapefruit, lemon, marjoram, and vetiver.

- **Benzoin:** anxiety, tension, nervousness, and stress. **Blends with:** orange, frankincense, bergamot, juniper, petit grain, coriander, lavender, lemon, myrrh, rose, and sandalwood.

- **Cedarwood:** acts as a sedative for anxiety and relaxation. **Blends with:** lavender, rose, neroli and rosemary, bergamot, benzoin, cypress, cinnamon, frankincense, juniper, jasmine, lemon and lime.

- **Frankincense:** acts as a sedative, and induces calm, relaxation, and mental peace. Promotes deep breathing that can help lower blood pressure. It awakens insight to support introspection and reduces stress, anger, and anxiety. **Blends with:** benzoin, bergamot, lavender, myrrh, lime, lemon, orange, pine, and sandalwood.

- **Geranium:** relieves tension and stress, works with the chakra to release toxins from the body, and helps to release negative memories. **Blends with:** all oils.

- **Jasmine:** produces confidence and optimism to alleviate depression. Induces calm, relaxation, relives headaches, and helps insomnia.

- **Blends with:** geranium, helichrysum, lemongrass, mandarin, Melissa, bergamot, frankincense, orange, palmarosa, rose, rosewood, sandalwood, and spearmint.

- **Wild Orange:** alleviates anxiety, boosts mood, and promotes a sense of happiness and wellbeing. Blends with: other citrus oils, bergamot, clove, cinnamon, and lavender.

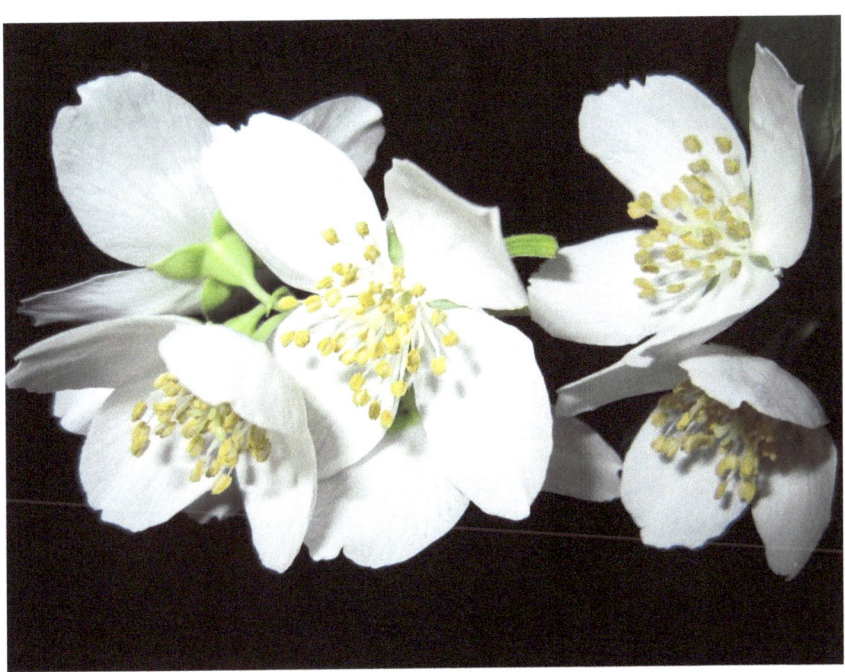

Make Your Own Essential Oils

The following recipes are for use in an aromatherapy diffuser. The number within the parentheses indicates the number of drops of each oil in the blend that is added to the water in a diffuser. Each recipe may be multiplied to create the desired amount of essential oil base while maintaining the ratios.

10 Synergistic Oil Recipes for Anxiety

1. Bergamot (2), Frankincense, (1) and Clary Sage (2)

2. Sandalwood (3) and Bergamot (2)

3. Bergamot (2), Lemon (2), Wild Orange (2), and Lavender (2)

4. Lavender (3) and Clary Sage (2)

5. Ylang-Ylang (1), Bergamot (2), Clary Sage (2), and Frankincense (2)

6. Lavender (3), Ylang Ylang (3), Basil (2), Geranium (2), and Grapefruit (2)

7. Rose (1), Vetiver (1), Lavender (1) and Mandarin (2)

8. Clary Sage (3), Frankincense (2), Geranium (3), Marjoram (3), and Orange (2)

9. Lavender (2), Geranium (2), and Sandalwood (2)

10. Bergamot (4), Eucalyptus (1), 2 drops Lavender (2) and peppermint (2)

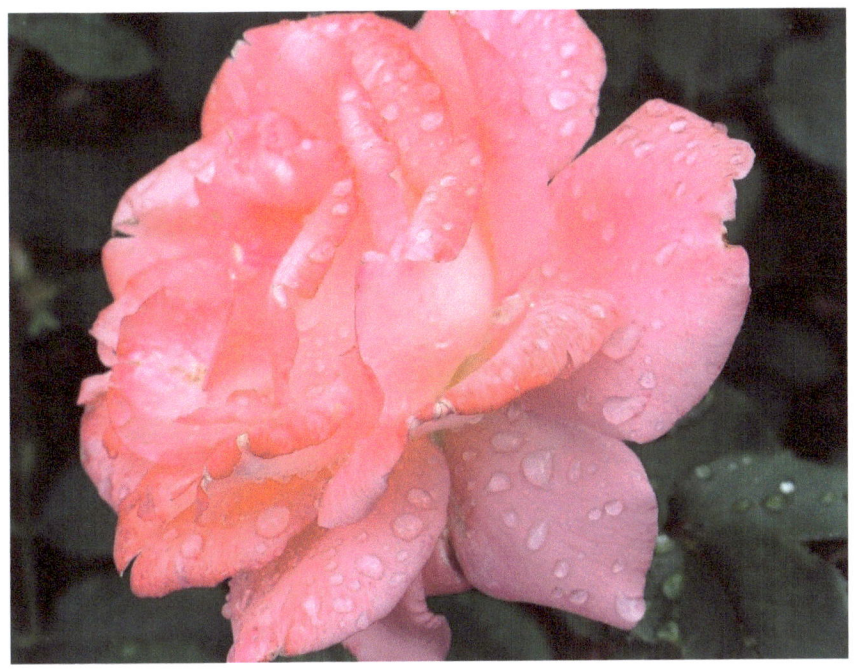

8 Synergistic Oil Recipes for Stress

1. Lemon (1), Lavender (1), and Clary Sage (3)

2. Lavender (2), Vetiver (1), and Roman Chamomile (2)

3. Geranium (1), Frankincense (1), and Bergamot (3)

4. Grapefruit (3), Ylang-Ylang (1), and Jasmine (1)

5. Roman Chamomile (4), Lavender (3), Clary Sage (2), Geranium (2), and 1 drop Ylang Ylang (1)

6. Lavender (4), Cedarwood (2), Orange (2), Ylang Ylang (1), and Vetiver (1)

7. Lavender (3), Geranium (3), Roman Chamomile (3), Clary Sage (2), and Ylang Ylang (3)

8. Lavender (4), Clary Sage (3), Ylang Ylang (2), and Marjoram (1)

How to Use Essential Oils for Aromatherapy

There are many ways to enjoy the benefits of essential oils. When selecting a method of application, the issue being treated must be considered along with the desired results.

- For example, creams, ointments, and gels work best for treating injuries like bruises and cuts.
- A massage oil works well for treating muscle aches and pains.
- If the primary purpose of the treatment is to shift a person's mood in some way, incense or a diffuser may be the best option.

Consider the following methods of delivery and choose the one best suited to the condition being treated as well as the person:

Diffuser

A diffuser disperses essential oils through the process of evaporation so their scent permeates a room or space. Diffusers can be very simple; for example, a tissue, on which a few drops of essential oils rest, becomes a diffuser when left on an out of the way surface for the oil to evaporate. Another option is to boil two cups of water and add up to ten drops of essential oil to it. The heat will cause the essential oil to evaporate more quickly to scent the room.

A Candle Diffuser also uses heat; the diffuser has a bottom portion to hold a tea light candle and a small bowl resting on top.

A few drops of essential oil are placed in the bowl which the lit tea light warms and causes the scent to permeate the room.

Hydrosols

Hydrosols are produced during the distillation process. They are the water that remains following the distillation process and contain the aromatic and therapeutic characteristics of the plant materials used to produce the essential oils. They are much less concentrated and in general may be used directly on the skin, mixed into other products for application or used alone as a body mist or cologne.

Incense

Plant gums, resins, and dried herbs are combined to make natural incense. If purchasing incense, make sure it does not contain synthetic materials. Also, be sure to burn the incense and place it somewhere the smoke drifts away from you. Inhaling incense smoke is on par with smoking.

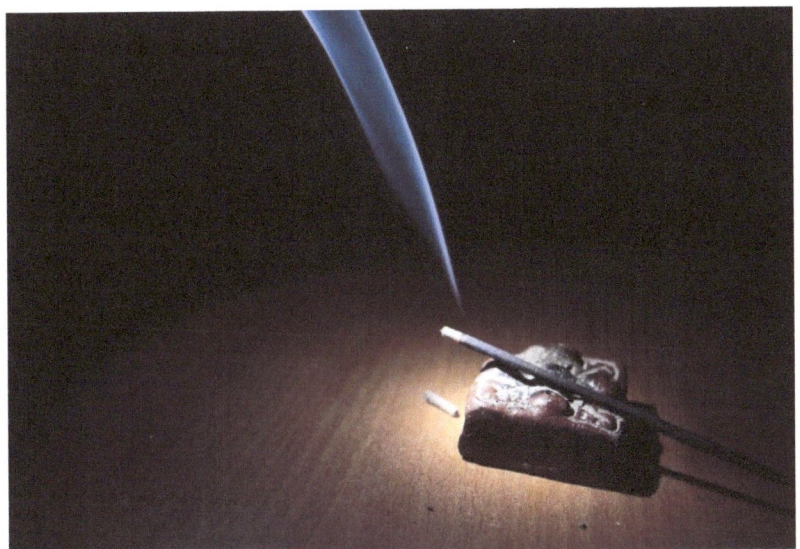

Massage Oils, Gels, and Creams

Pre-blended aromatherapy massage oils, gels, and creams may be applied following a shower or bath while the skin is damp. It aids in applying the preparation evenly and the absorption of the treatment into the skin.

You may also mix your own. It is always best to dilute the essential oils in a carrier oil to disperse the oils and lessen their concentration as they can burn when applied directly to the skin.

Ratios: Generally, 2 drops of essential oil should be added per one teaspoon of carrier oil, but always follow any given recipe as instructed. 1 to 2 ounces of carrier oil is enough for one full body massage.

Best Carrier Oils:

- Canola oil – great for massage, absorbs into the skin easily, light and odorless.

- Sunflower oil – Ideal for massage and body lotions and rich in Vitamin E
- Sweet Almond oil – good as a massage oil; loaded with protein; absorbs into the skin rapidly; odorless
- Jojoba oil – Super nourishing and softens dry skin.
- Avocado oil – softens skin.
- Grapeseed oil – Lightweight, and works great for massage and facials.
- Hazelnut oil – Contains minerals, proteins and vitamins and makes for an excellent carrier oil for facials blends.
- Olive oil – Olive oil works great for most recipes, and extra virgin olive oil has the most nutrients.
- Hazelnut oil – Contains vital proteins and vitamins.
- Safflower oil – good for softening the skin; it's a light-to-medium weight oil.
- Evening Primrose oil – contains essential antioxidants, and can prolong shelf life of other oils.
- Castor oil – good for sealing in moisture; a heavy oil that seals and protects
- Corn oil – a medium weight oil that has minerals and vitamins for skin health
- Sesame oil – Contains high levels of Vitamin E, proteins and minerals so it's really good for the skin.
- Soy oil – Rich in Vitamin E.

Bath Oils and Bath Salts

While essential oils may be added directly to bath water, which is agitated before entering, using bath oils and bath salts are a safer option. Essential oils will eventually separate from the water to float on the surface, which presents the risk of burning the skin while soaking in the bath. Bath oils and baths salts act as carriers to ensure the essential oils remain diluted and dispersed in the bath water.

Aromatherapy Candles

Aromatherapy candles disperse essential oils through the air from candles, if choosing this method be sure to get a high quality candle that notes the use of essential oils and natural wax ingredients, like soy.

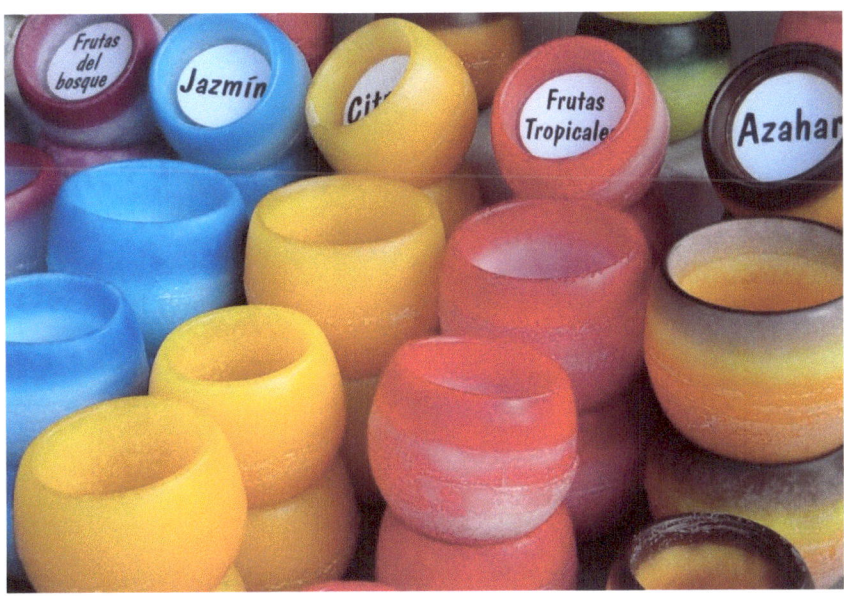

Satchel

You can enjoy the therapeutic and relaxing effects of flowers and plants when going to sleep by placing a satchel under or near your pillow. Dried lavender works great.

As with any therapy practice, educate yourself about the pros and cons of including it in your treatment regimen. Seek out the counsel of the appropriate medical practitioner and an aromatherapist.

They can evaluate your medical history and make the appropriate recommendations for your successful use of aromatherapy if no contraindications, allergies, or drug interactions exist.

In the End ... Its Up to You!

Stress kills! This is a fact, and we live in a fast paced, "go get em" world that is full of stress. While some suffer intermittent bouts of stress, others live in a chronic state of stress that can have a serious effect on their health.

TAKE THE TIME FOR TRUE RELAXATION!

Stillness...

Calm...

Quite...

It is critical to your health to find the time or more precisely make the time to relax!

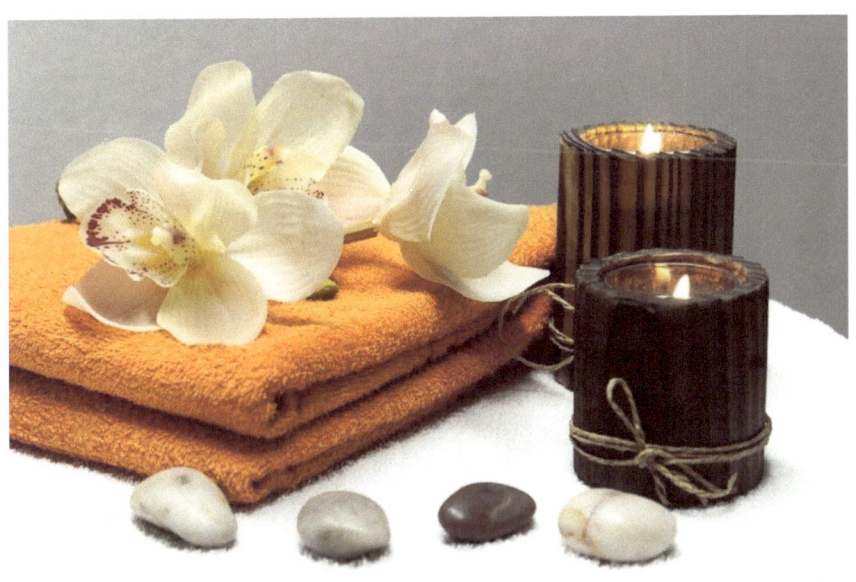

Many options elicit the relaxation response. Some of the best are yoga, Tai Chi, Qi Gong, progressive relaxation, breathing exercises, mediation, and aromatherapy.

Aromatherapy as a management tool for stress and anxiety works best in conjunction with other therapies, though it is also a hands-free solution that can be implemented any time, such as with a diffuser on your desk pumping out lavender that you will absorb while working.

Other alternative therapies like yoga, meditation, and progressive relaxation benefit from the use of aromatherapy during their practice. The aromatherapy component assists with inducing the desired calm and relaxed mental and physical states that can support a positive mood AND overall health and wellness.

NOW GO AND RELAX!

About the Author

Besides my own writing and publishing, I also ghostwrite ebooks, reports, articles, blogs and do Kindle conversions for my clients on a variety of topics.

Today my wife and I live in Gold Canyon, AZ, where you'll find me happily sitting in my office typing away on my laptop as I work on my next book or ghostwriting project . . . that is if we are not traveling on a cruise ship - our new-found mode of travel.

If you like this book, please leave a review of it. To see more of my published works on Createspace, just search "Ron Kness" (without quotes) on their website.

www.ingramcontent.com/pod-product-compliance
Lightning Source LLC
Chambersburg PA
CBHW050850290526
45792CB00002B/593